The Mother Tree

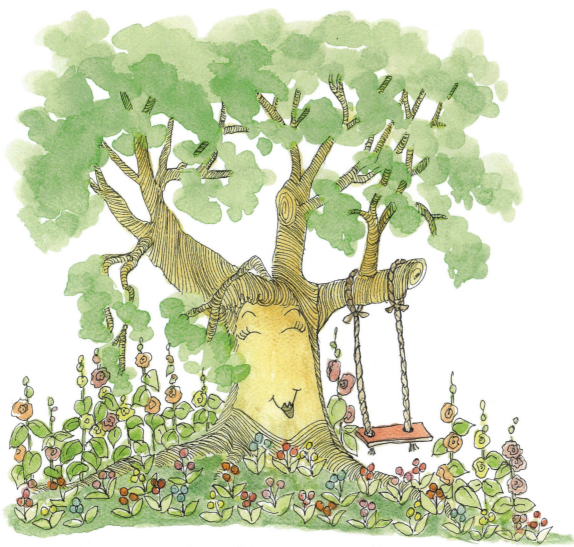

authored & illustrated by jc west

Conception of this book:
Korakia Pensione
(under the lemon tree)
March 1993, Palm Springs, CA

Artwork and Revisions:
(under the Queen Mother Tree)
1993-1995, Pasadena, CA

Finished for Publication:
(under the palm trees)
2012-2016, Rancho Mirage, CA

Technical Design:
Criss Ittermann, Eclectic Tech, LLC
(under the maple trees)
2016, Middletown, NY

Copyright 2016 by Jan West Castro.

All rights reserved. No part of this book may be reproduced or transmitted in any form by any means, electronic or mechanical, including photocopying and recording, or by any information storage and retrieval system.

Requests for permission should be made in writing to:
Jan West Castro
jan.jcwest@gmail.com
Rancho Mirage, California

THE MOTHER TREE is a trademark of jc west aka Jan West Castro.
All illustrations property of jc west aka Jan West Castro.

Manufactured in the United States of America.
To order more jc west book titles go to: www.amazon.com

This book is dedicated to the trees I have befriended and grown with.

The Eucalyptus Tree at my grandparent's home. Its beautiful bark fascinated me.
— Wilmington, California —

The big old grove Walnut Tree in our brand-new 1950's tract home.
She was my horse...we "rode" far and wide.
— Tarzana, California —

The brilliant fall Maple Trees and the nostalgic smell of a burning leaves.
— Birmingham, Michigan —

The Banana and Mango Trees so indigenous yet so exotic!
— Santa Maria, Puerto Rico —

The Sycamore seedling that grew to be huge.
— San Diego, California —

The lone Avocado Tree, so generous with her delicious fruit.
— San Gabriel, California —

The Live Oak Trees, one with a rope swing hanging from her strong limb.
The Pepper Tree that cradled our daughters' tree house.
The amazing lavender Jacarandas that still grace the city.
— Pasadena, California —

The desert Palm Trees that sway, sparkle and shine in the late afternoon light.
— Coachella Valley, California —

The Giant Redwood Trees to whom I have always felt a very special connection.
— Northern California —

And lastly...the most queenly tree of them all. A magnificent camphor, a true
'MOTHER TREE' located at 207 S. Fair Oaks Ave., behind Happy Trails Catering.
Lunch in her shade!
— Pasadena, California —

— You have all enhanced and blessed my life. Truly!

Thank you, Jan West Castro (aka jc west)

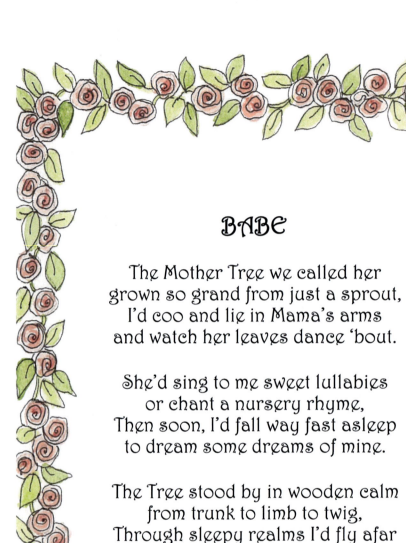

BABE

The Mother Tree we called her
grown so grand from just a sprout,
I'd coo and lie in Mama's arms
and watch her leaves dance 'bout.

She'd sing to me sweet lullabies
or chant a nursery rhyme,
Then soon, I'd fall way fast asleep
to dream some dreams of mine.

The Tree stood by in wooden calm
from trunk to limb to twig,
Through sleepy realms I'd fly afar
and wonder 'bout being big.

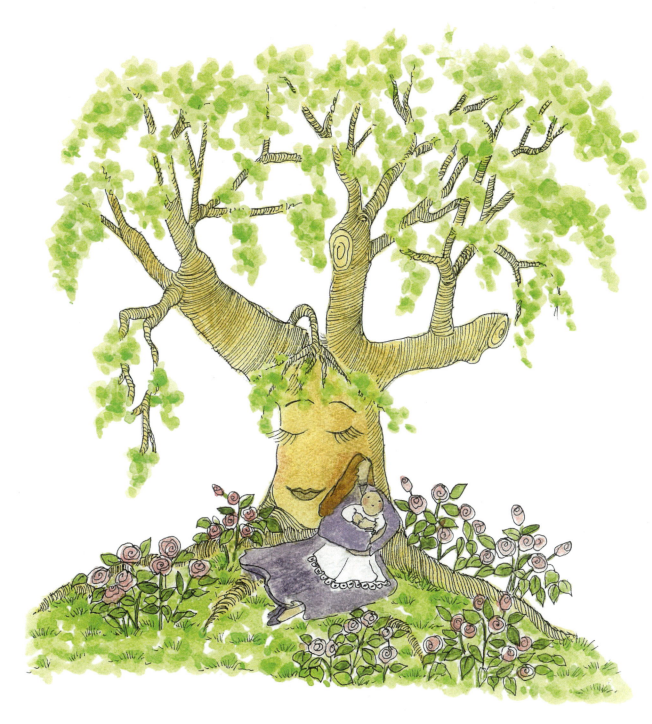

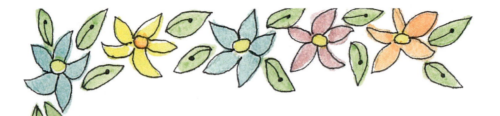

TODDLER

Then one day Daddy gathered up
a ladder and some rope,
A boost upon his shoulders and...
we headed up the slope.

There, Mother Tree was waiting,
with a limb saved just for me,
We hung a swing so I could fly...
and squeal with wide-eyed glee.

I'd fly up to the sky so fast
and down with lightning speed,
Then up again and higher still,
"Don't ever stop!" I'd plead.

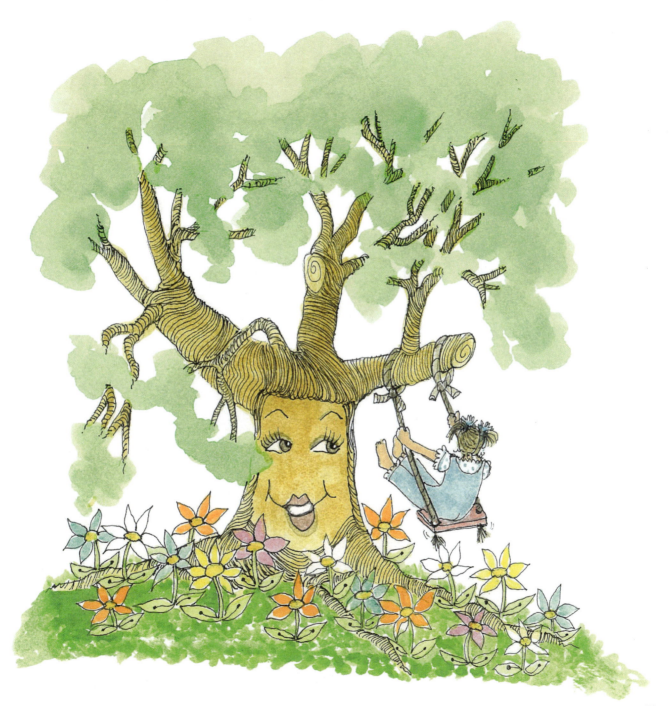

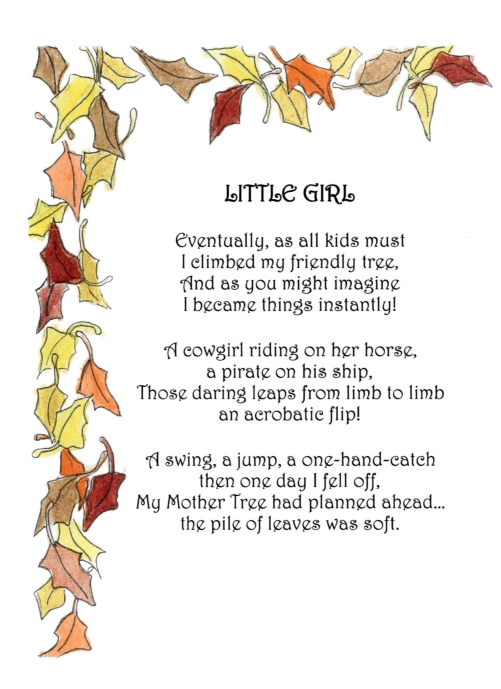

LITTLE GIRL

Eventually, as all kids must
I climbed my friendly tree,
And as you might imagine
I became things instantly!

A cowgirl riding on her horse,
a pirate on his ship,
Those daring leaps from limb to limb
an acrobatic flip!

A swing, a jump, a one-hand-catch
then one day I fell off,
My Mother Tree had planned ahead...
the pile of leaves was soft.

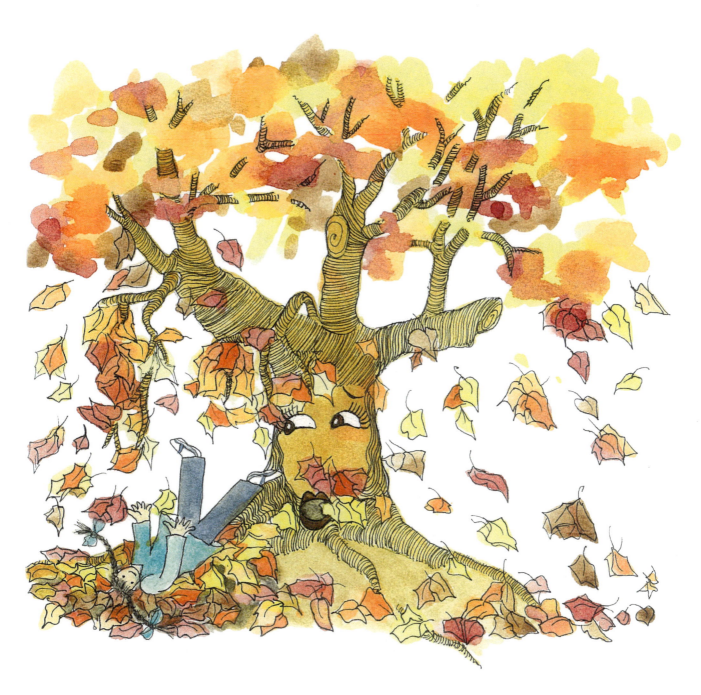

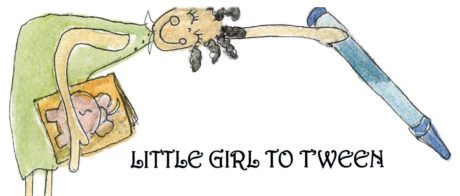

LITTLE GIRL TO T'WEEN

As seasons passed I played with dolls
and color books and friends,
And wanting to be grown-up wondered...
"When will childhood end?"

My Tree knew that this time of life
holds treasures rich as gold,
a 'time of plenty'... mem-or-ies
to dwell upon when old.

From babe to girl to t'ween I grew
with love and feeling free,
There also were those shady days
...It's how I be'came me.

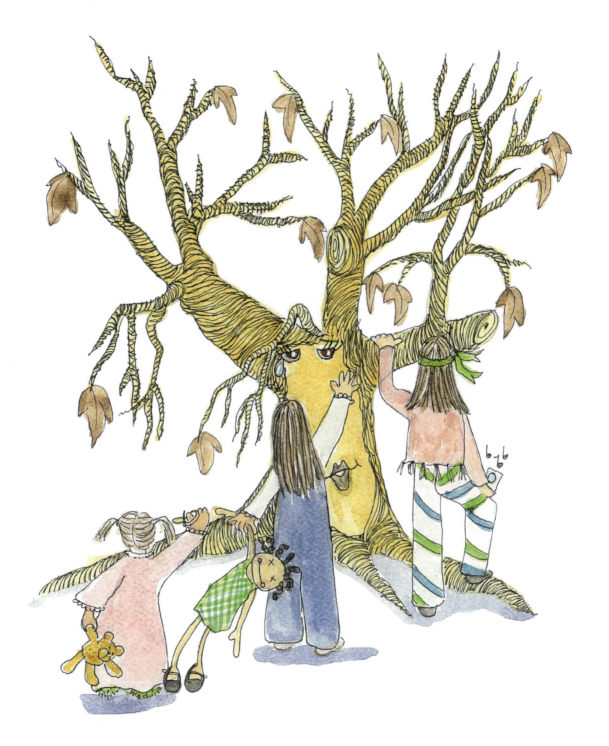

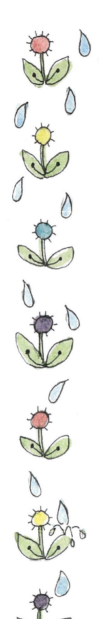

TEEN

My Mother Tree was witness when
my lips had their first kiss,
And stood there mum and silent when,
a romance went amiss.

With arms around her barky breast
a girl could have a cry,
Quite un-like everybody else
She never had to pry.

I've often wished that I could give
as much as she gives me,
It's odd to think that some would say,
"It's just a big old tree!"

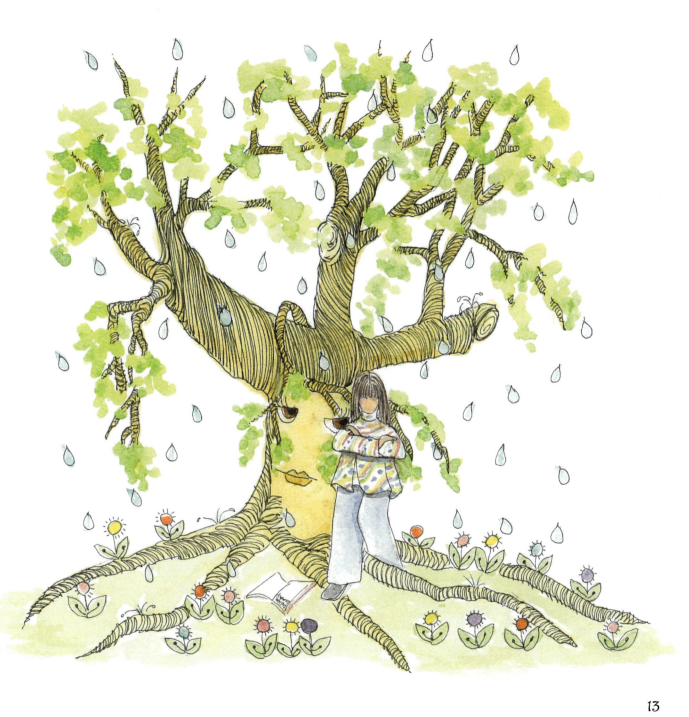

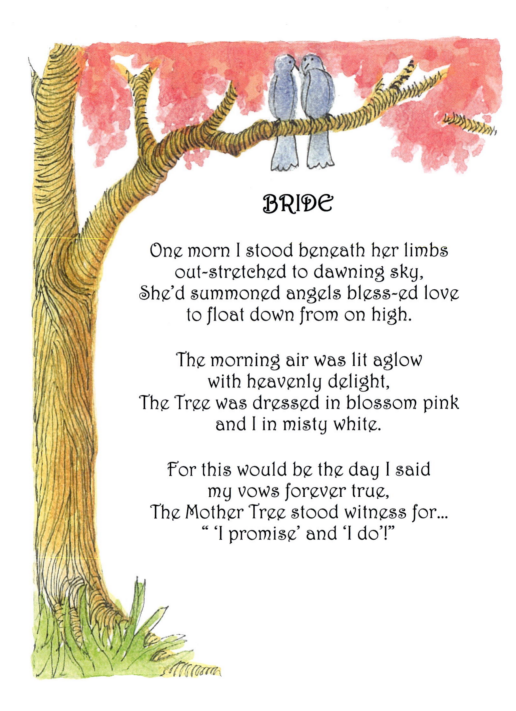

BRIDE

One morn I stood beneath her limbs
out-stretched to dawning sky,
She'd summoned angels bless-ed love
to float down from on high.

The morning air was lit aglow
with heavenly delight,
The Tree was dressed in blossom pink
and I in misty white.

For this would be the day I said
my vows forever true,
The Mother Tree stood witness for...
" 'I promise' and 'I do'!"

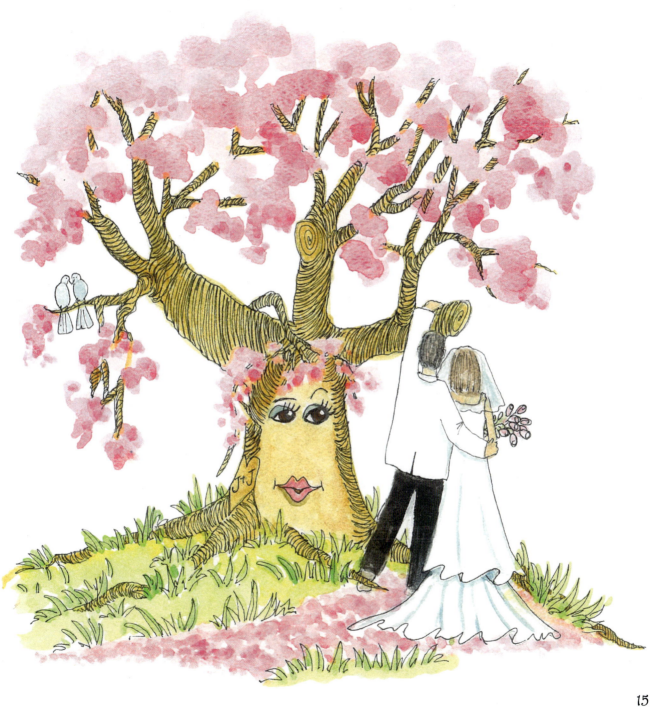

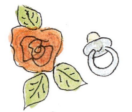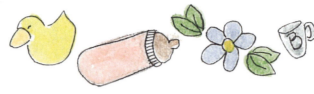

MOTHER TO BE

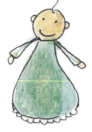

The past few years have spun and blurred
We've worked so hard to build,
A life and nest for little ones
and with that news...we're thrilled!

As tiny seed grows deep within
a miracle for sure,
I rest beneath The Mother Tree
and dream of babes demure.

She's watched this scene unfold before
fulfillment of desire,
And knows there is such bliss in store
as well as...tests by fire.

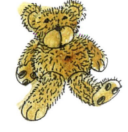

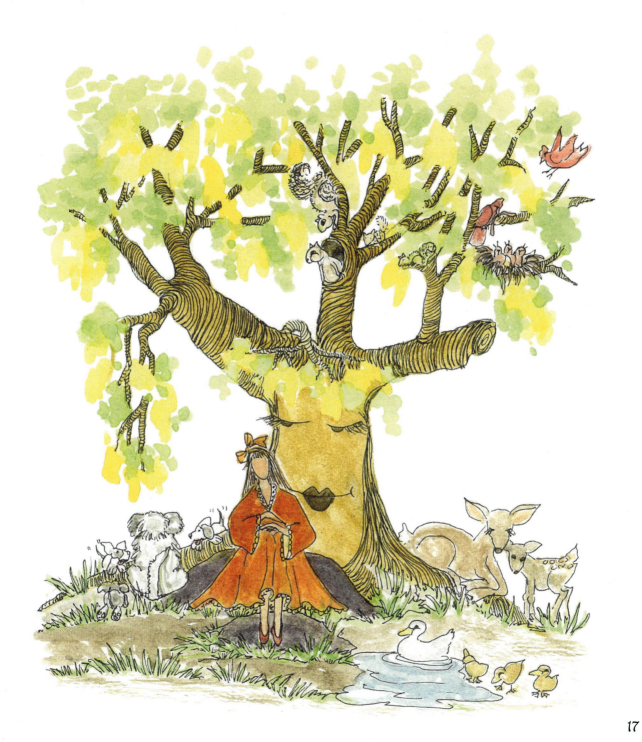

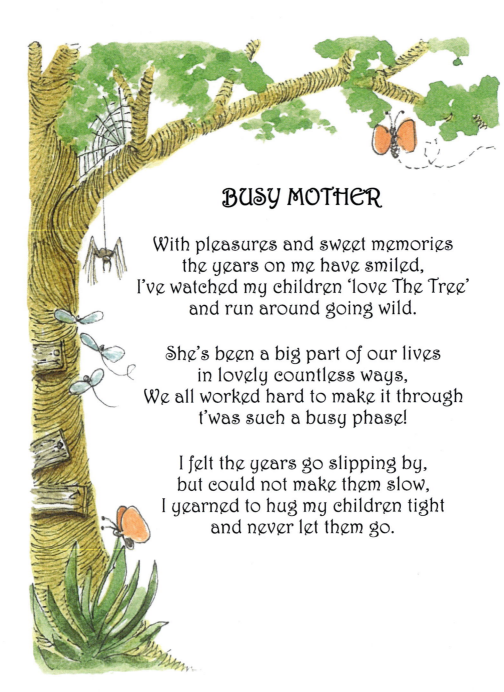

BUSY MOTHER

With pleasures and sweet memories
the years on me have smiled,
I've watched my children 'love The Tree'
and run around going wild.

She's been a big part of our lives
in lovely countless ways,
We all worked hard to make it through
t'was such a busy phase!

I felt the years go slipping by,
but could not make them slow,
I yearned to hug my children tight
and never let them go.

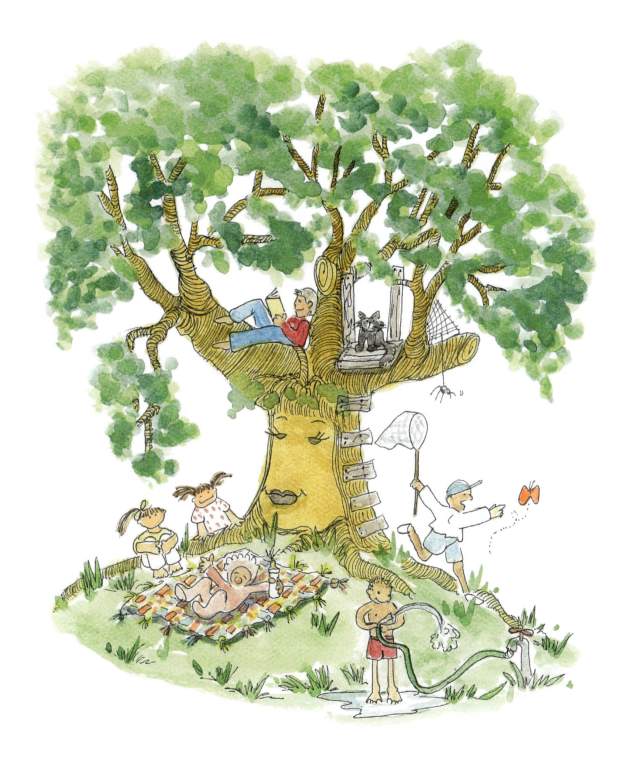

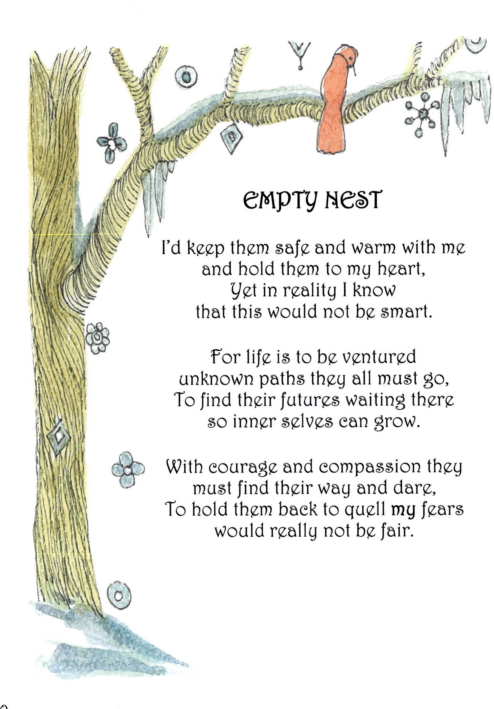

EMPTY NEST

I'd keep them safe and warm with me
and hold them to my heart,
Yet in reality I know
that this would not be smart.

For life is to be ventured
unknown paths they all must go,
To find their futures waiting there
so inner selves can grow.

With courage and compassion they
must find their way and dare,
To hold them back to quell **my** fears
would really not be fair.

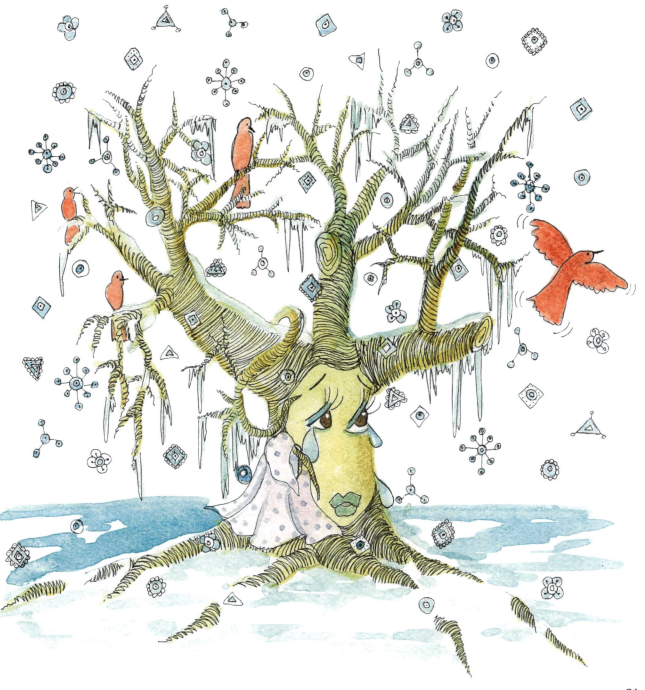

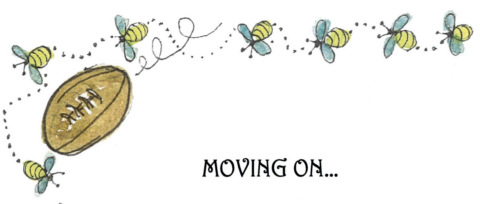

MOVING ON...

Our big old house is empty now
once filled with active kids,
And jars chuck-full of critter things,
"What's happened to those lids?!"

So many dogs and cats and rats
and frogs and snakes and such,
Amazing all the goings on
it really was too much!

The Tree, my love and I look back
and truly must confess,
We loved it all and would not trade
but, "Goodness, that was stress!"

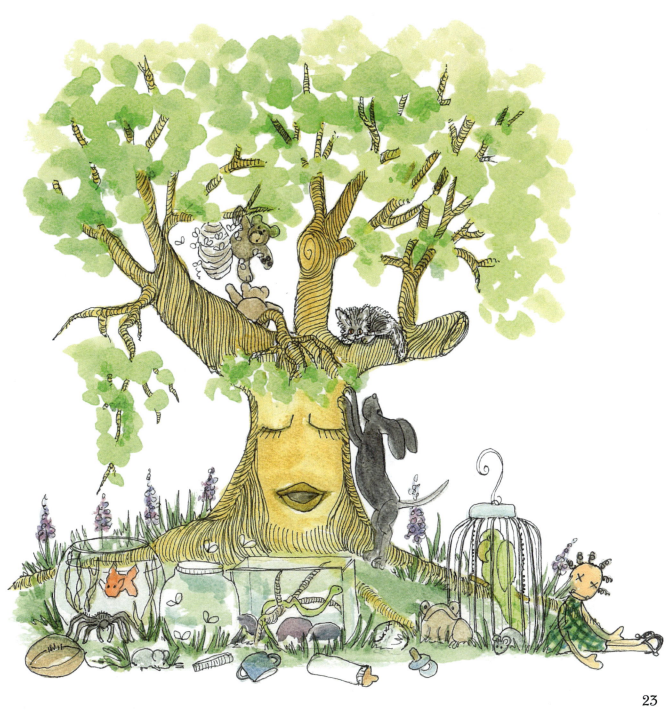

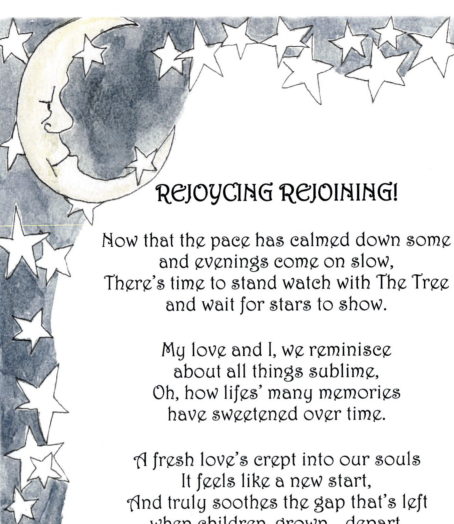

REJOYCING REJOINING!

Now that the pace has calmed down some
and evenings come on slow,
There's time to stand watch with The Tree
and wait for stars to show.

My love and I, we reminisce
about all things sublime,
Oh, how lifes' many memories
have sweetened over time.

A fresh love's crept into our souls
It feels like a new start,
And truly soothes the gap that's left
when children, grown... depart.

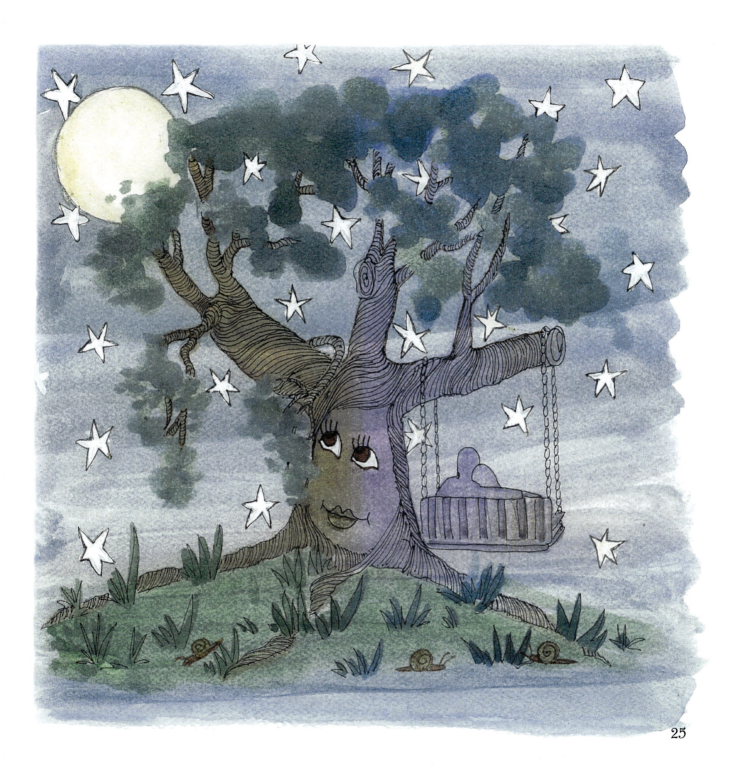

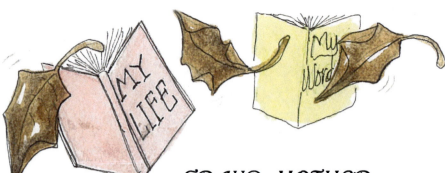

GRAND...MOTHER

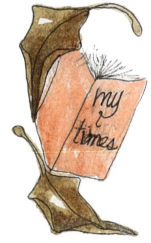

The days seem somehow longer now
a peace surrounds my being,
I'm taking time to listen
and to "see" what I am seeing.

The grandkids come to visit us
and bring such lively fun,
With kisses, hugs and storybooks
and games 'til day is done.

The Mother Trees' example of
just being their lovingly,
Is what I give these little ones
with me...they're free to be!

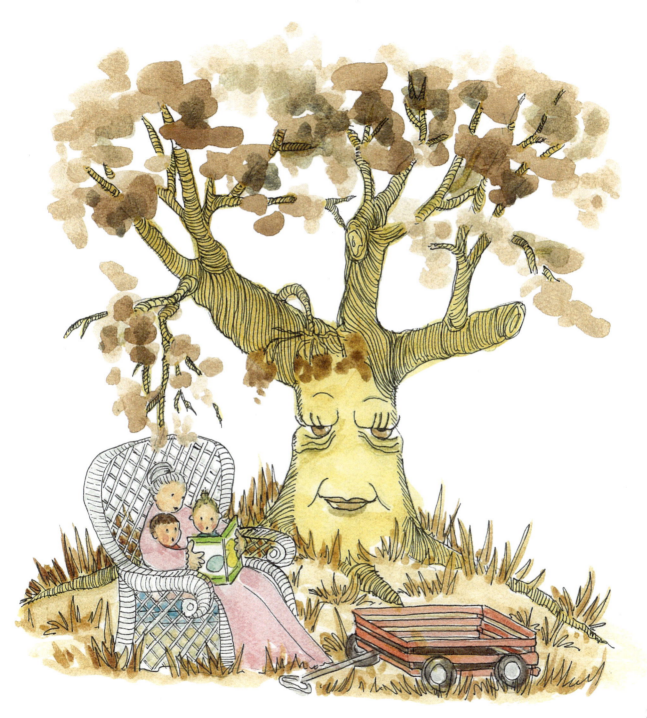

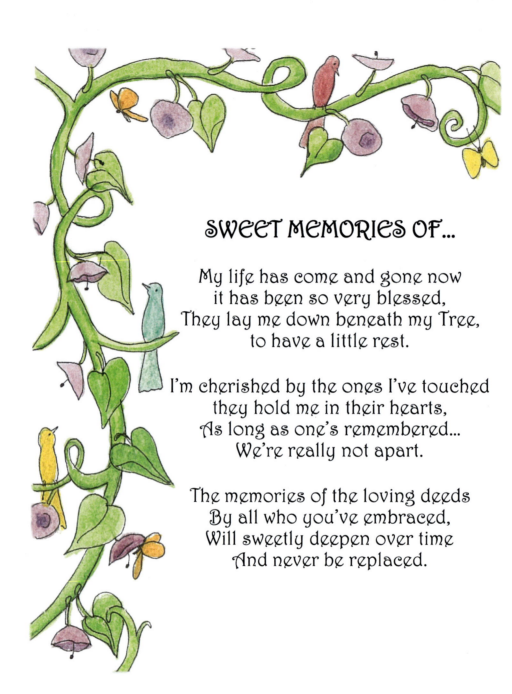

SWEET MEMORIES OF...

My life has come and gone now
it has been so very blessed,
They lay me down beneath my Tree,
to have a little rest.

I'm cherished by the ones I've touched
they hold me in their hearts,
As long as one's remembered...
We're really not apart.

The memories of the loving deeds
By all who you've embraced,
Will sweetly deepen over time
And never be replaced.

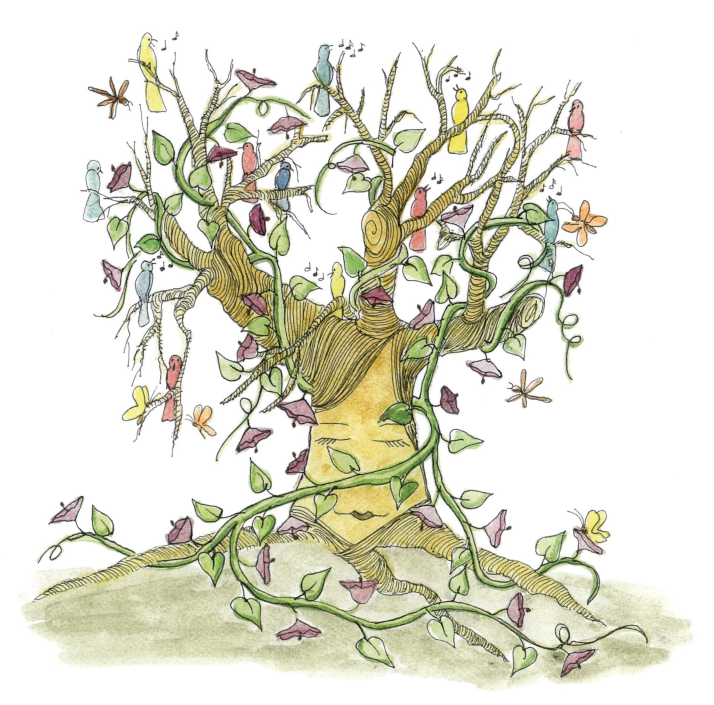

WE ALL ARE MOTHER TREES

In truth we all are Mother Trees
how meaningful this phrase:
"One needn't to have given birth
to touch in moth'ring ways."

By thoughtfulness and tenderness
a husband, child or friend,
Can shower you with 'acts of love'...
a mother would extend.

When "Mother Trees" surround you with
their warm arboreal light,
You've somehow got the feeling that...
things really are all right.

God bless the trees and mothers for
their goodness freely spent.
And make a vow you'll pass it on...
so **much** their love has meant.

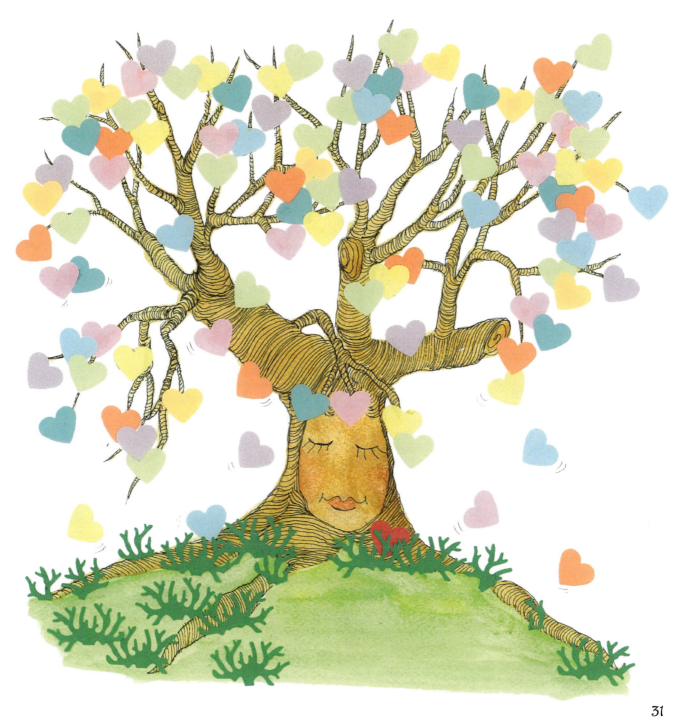

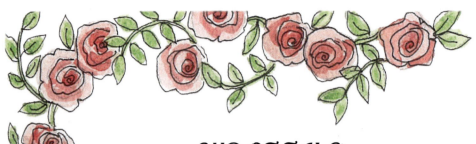

END OF TALE

It's not too late to find
a Mother Tree to call your own,
She's standing there within your sight
just look and you'll be shown.

You've found a true friend, that will be
awaiting any cue,
Of how she may, in any way
be 'specially there for you!

In recognition limbs will sway
she'll quiver to her leaves,
You'll only need an open heart...
and "be one who believes!"

So this, alas, is end of tale
from babe to womanhood,
About a life long friendship with...
a lovely 'being of wood'.

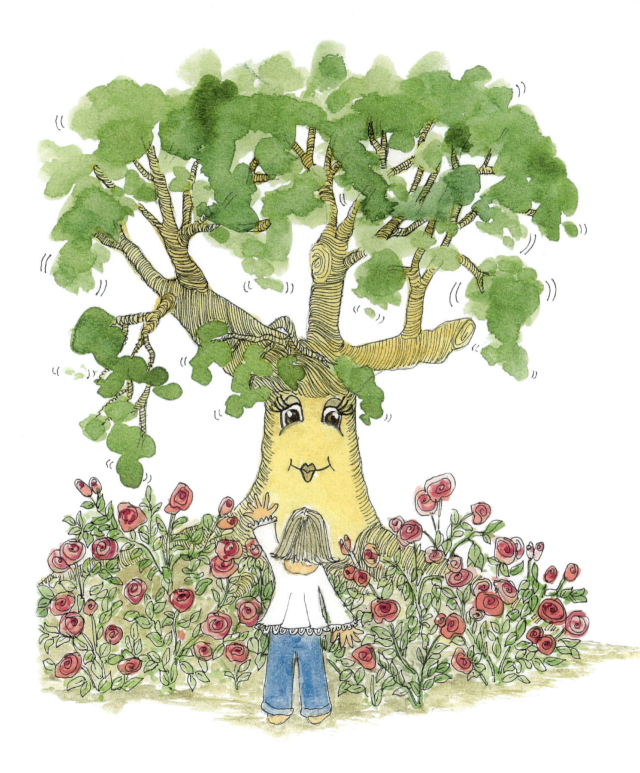

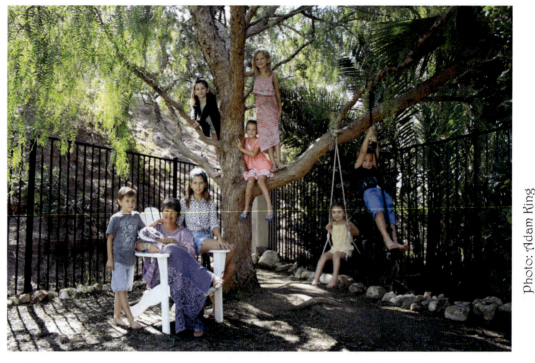

THE MOTHER TREE, ME (JANJAN) AND MY EIGHT GRANDCHILDREN

In the King's Mother Tree: Gillian Gehring (9) and Vivyanna & Gloryanna McLinn (8 1/2 & 10 1/2).
On the Chair: Cayson & Sicily Jaye King (7 1/2 & 2 days old), JanJan and Jorja Gehring (11).
On the Swings: Julianna McLinn (4) and Brooks King (5).

Imagine how my heart leapt when, for the first time, I walked into the back yard of my daughters' new home and saw this pepper tree. It was February 2012, over twenty years past the time I first began conceiving of the illustrations for The Mother Tree book. There, in the far corner, stood a perfect replica of the tree I had envisioned and watercolored for my story. She seemed to be expectantly waiting with 'limbs open wide'...ready to welcome a young mother and her family into her yard and heart. Now, all of my eight grandchildren know her.

May there be many happy years of experiencing life and...growing together!

P.S. When I go for a visit I always make it a point to say, "Hello." and give the tree a little hug.

About the Author & Illustrator

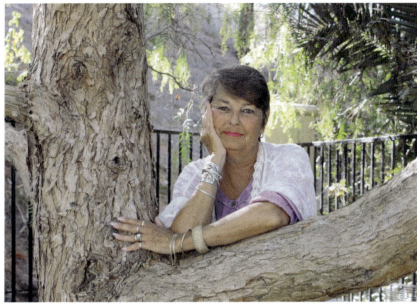

Photo: Adam King

Jan West Castro (aka jc west)

I am......known to many as JanJan, Jay's wife of 45+ loving years, the mother to three adored daughters, mother-in-awe of three great guys, grandmother to eight dear ones: two grandsons and six granddaughters. Ages eleven to new born.

I am also... a watercolorist, a verse writer, a petter of three kitties, a legacy leaver, a flower gardener, a crafter, feminine-ist*, a 'Power of Now' practitioner, a Capricorn, a memory maker, a book writer**, a beach sitter, a frister***, an observer of life, an admirer and believer in Father God and Mother Nature, a hearth and home designer, a clothes horse, an avid Pinterest user, a communer, one who crochets, a student of metaphysics, a champagne sipper, a candle lighter, AND... a life-long dreamer of becoming a future recipient of the Caldacott Medal.****

*as opposed to being a feminist.
**see amazon.com for my book on relationships titled, Puppy Love 101.
***a friend you get to choose to be like a sister.
****recognition of year's most distinguished American picture book for children.

Trees
by Joyce Kilmer (1913)

I think that I shall never see
A poem lovely as a tree.

A tree whose hungry mouth is prest
Against the earth's sweet flowing breast;

A tree that looks at God all day,
And lifts her leafy arms to pray;

A tree that may in Summer wear
A nest of robins in her hair;

Upon whose bosom snow has lain;
Who intimately lives with rain.

Poems are made by fools like me,
But only God can make a tree.

Made in the USA
Coppell, TX
24 January 2023

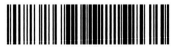